The Apply2Medicine Guide to Writing your Medical School Personal Statement:
Your Way, Successfully

Dr Tony Edgar MB BS, MSc, FFPH
Mr Matt Green BSc, MPhil

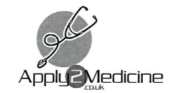

ISBN: 978-0-9556746-0-0

Published by Apply2 Ltd
Chelsea House, Chelsea Street, Northgate,
Nottingham, NG7 7HN.

Prepared by:
York Publishing Services Ltd
64 Hallfield Road
Layerthorpe
York
YO31 7ZQ
Tel: 01904 431213 Website: www.yps-publishing.co.uk

Contents

About the authors

Tony Edgar, MB BS, MSc, FFPH

Tony qualified in Medicine from Newcastle University in 1971. After working as a principal in general practice in the north-east of England, he undertook specialty training in public health in Manchester. In 1994 he was appointed Medical Director of the Fosse Health NHS Trust in Leicestershire; in 2002 he was elected Fellow of the Faculty of Public Health of the Royal Colleges of Physicians of the United Kingdom.

Matt Green, BSc, MPhil

After completing his BSc in Biochemistry, Matt went on to complete an MPhil at the Royal Marsden Hospital in Sutton, Surrey. This involved working closely with medical professionals on a number of projects developing novel drugs for the treatment of ovarian cancer. For the last three years Matt has worked closely with prospective medical students assisting them in their applications and subsequent interview preparations.

Matt and Tony are keen to share their respective experiences in supporting applicants to medical school. Working alongside other professional colleagues in Apply2Medicine, they provide advice, up to date guidance, and support with regard to the preparation of candidates' Personal Statements, selection interviews and entrance examinations. If after reading this book you are keen to obtain further guidance or assistance, please visit our website www.apply2medicine.co.uk where we will be happy to help you.

Acknowledgements

We would like to thank all of the prospective medical students we have supported in the last three years; they have enabled the writing of this book to become a reality.

Special thanks also go to Nicola and to Safia for their ongoing support and advice.

Preface

"What is Medicine?

Medicine offers a broad range of careers from general practice to the specialties of hospital practice and to medical research. Medicine is an applied science, but it is equally about dealing sympathetically and effectively with individuals, whether they be patients or colleagues. Medicine increasingly poses difficult ethical dilemmas, and above all, medicine is constantly and rapidly developing and providing a stimulating challenge to practitioners and medical scientists alike."

Oxford University website: June 2007

This informative guide is intended to help applicants to medical schools in the United Kingdom submit an effective, compelling Personal Statement. It seeks to assist school leaver, graduate and mature applicants alike, as well as parents and teachers. Please use this guide alongside advice provided by your school or college, from the Universities and College Admissions Service, and assistance offered by the medical schools themselves.

This guide includes examples from real and fictitious 'Personal Statements' in order to illustrate certain key principles. It is vitally important that you see them as they are – illustrative examples.

The most important aspect of your Personal Statement is that it is written by, and is about, you!

Chapter 1

Applying to a medical school in the United Kingdom: The process

In 2005 there were over twenty two thousand applications to study Medicine and Dentistry in the United Kingdom. Across the country, there are on average around 5 applications for each medical school place on offer.

There are three steps in this application process:

- Sitting the appropriate entrance examination where applicable
  (Examinations take place between June and October in the year before successful candidates begin their medical studies.)

- Submitting a university application which includes the Personal Statement (Mid-October deadline)

- Attending a selection interview when applicable (Interviews take place between October and the following June depending upon the medical school)

Medical school entrance examinations

An increasing number of medical schools require candidates to complete an entrance examination before submitting their actual application. It is therefore important to determine as soon as possible whether or not the medical schools to which you intend to apply require you to sit an entrance examination. Those in current use are based upon an aptitude format assessing a number of different criteria. The aim of these tests is to aid the application process by ensuring that appropriate attitude, mental competence and professional qualities are specifically considered. Presently there are three examination formats in use in the UK:

- United Kingdom Clinical Aptitude Test (UKCAT)
- Biomedical Admissions Test (BMAT)
- Graduate Medical Schools Admissions Test (GAMSAT)

The closing dates for these tests differ and we advise you to consult the relevant websites listed in the following sections for more information.

UKCAT

The UKCAT aptitude test was formally adopted in 2006 by twenty three of the medical schools in the UK. The test is designed to assist admissions tutors towards selecting candidates who possess the desired mental abilities, approaches and attributes of successful medical students and practising doctors.

The test sets out to examine the following five qualities:

- Verbal reasoning
- Quantitative reasoning
- Abstract reasoning
- Decision analysis
- Non-cognitive analysis

For more information visit:

www.ukcat.org.uk
www.apply2medicine.co.uk/ukcat

BMAT

The BMAT aptitude test is currently used by a number of medical schools, including Cambridge, Oxford, Imperial College and University College, London.

The test covers three sections:

- Section 1 This evaluates generic skills which are important for effective undergraduate study. These include complex problem solving techniques, evaluating balanced arguments, and the ability to analyse data.
- Section 2 This is restricted to topics in mathematics and science
- Section 3 This normally comprises a short essay

For more information and advice regarding the BMAT test visit:

www.bmat.org.uk
www.apply2medicine.co.uk/bmat

GAMSAT

The GAMSAT aptitude test was developed by the Australian Council for Medical Research and is specifically used in the consideration of graduate applicants to medical schools. Among the UK universities which use the GAMSAT test are the University of Wales and Nottingham University.

The GAMSAT test evaluates:

- Practical experience, attributes and skills
- Knowledge and implementation of concepts in basis science
- Problem solving, critical thinking and writing skills

For more information and advice regarding the GAMSAT test visit:

www.apply2medicine.co.uk/gamsat

The UCAS Application

As the competition for medical school places continues to increase, the need for a clear, engaging and well-structured university application is paramount. The Universities and Colleges Admission Service (UCAS) mediate applications made to universities in the United Kingdom through an online system (for more information visit www.ucas.com). If you are at school or college, the application process will be co-ordinated by the head of post-16 education and you will be provided with login details and instructions on how to proceed. If you are applying as a graduate or mature student not currently in full time education, you can register with UCAS directly in order to submit your application.

You cannot apply directly to a UK medical school to study Medicine. All applications must be made via UCAS using the somewhat daunting 'UCAS Application Form' which is now in electronic format. Although the paper-based 'UCAS Form' is not commonly used now for applications to medical school, the electronic application process still requires all of the information that would have been previously submitted. Accordingly, the electronic UCAS form requires you to enter your personal details, your course choices, your predicted or actual grades, your Reference and your Personal Statement.

When considering an application to medical school, the admissions tutors place particular emphasis upon your entrance examination result (where applicable), academic performance, your Reference and your Personal Statement. Indeed, some medical schools currently make offers to students based solely on their applications without conducting any interviews.

At present, the medical school Personal Statement must be completed within 4000 characters. It is also important to note that when entering the Personal Statement onto the UCAS system, any formatting- such as underlining, italics or bolding- will be lost.

So, **YOUR** UCAS Personal Statement is **YOUR** key opportunity to convince medical school admissions tutors that **YOU** are an exceptional candidate and that they should offer **YOU** a place at their medical school over other applicants.

It is vital that you make your comments clearly and compellingly, so that the admissions tutors become really keen to meet you and find out more about this special, unique person that you are!

Applying to study different subjects

Currently, candidates applying to study Medicine are restricted to applying to four medical schools in a calendar year whereas applicants for degree subjects other than Medicine are invited to apply to six universities. Accordingly, applicants to study Medicine are also able to apply for two other non-medical courses, such as Pharmacy or Biomedical Sciences. However it is important to remember that within each candidate's application, only one Personal Statement can be submitted.

It is the advice of the authors, based upon their practical experience, that candidates seeking to study Medicine should write their Personal Statement wholly with the aim of gaining acceptance to study Medicine. Any attempt to incorporate other course choices would be inadvisable; such an approach would almost certainly reduce the strength of the Personal Statement.

Key message

Make sure that you first make contact with UCAS, the entrance examinations websites, and the medical schools themselves in order to find out *exactly* what you need to do when applying to study Medicine. Attending university 'Open Days' is especially valuable; you have the chance then to ask questions directly.

Chapter 2

What kind of students do medical schools want?

The Council of Heads of Medical Schools, in consultation with the Department of Health and British Medical Association, have produced a statement setting out guiding principles for the selection and admission of students to medical schools.

These are:

1. **Selection for medical school implies selection for the medical profession.**
   A degree in Medicine confirms academic achievement and in normal circumstances entitles the new graduate to be provisionally registered by the General Medical Council.

2. The selection process attempts to identify the core academic and non-academic qualities of a doctor:

   − **Honesty, integrity** and an ability to **recognise one's own limitations** and those of others, are central to the practice of medicine.
   − Other key attributes include having **good communication** and **listening skills**, an ability **to make decisions under pressure**, and to **remain calm and cope with stress.**

- Doctors must have an understanding of **teamwork** and respect for the contributions of others. Desirable characteristics include **curiosity, creativity, initiative, flexibility** and **leadership.**

3. A high level of academic attainment will be expected. **Understanding science is core to the understanding of medicine,** but medical schools generally encourage diversity in subjects studied by candidates.

4. The practice of medicine requires the highest standards of **professional** and **personal conduct.** Put simply, some students will not be suited to a career in medicine and it is in the interests of the student and the public that they should not be admitted to medical school.

5. The practice of medicine requires the highest standards of **professional competence.** However, a history of serious ill health or disability will not jeopardize a career in medicine unless the condition impinges upon professional fitness to practise.

6. Candidates should demonstrate some **understanding of what a career in medicine involves** and their suitability for a **caring profession.**
Medical schools expect candidates to have had some relevant experience in health or related areas. Indeed, some medical schools stipulate a defined minimum period of relevant work experience.

7. The **primary duty of care is to patients.** All applicants to medical schools will be expected to understand the importance of this principle.

8. Failure to declare information that has a material influence on a student's fitness to practise may lead to termination of their medical course.

Clearly, it is important that you consult the websites of the medical schools to which you intend to apply in order to learn of any specific requirements they are seeking.

University education is also expensive. For every medical student who drops out, there are financial implications to the university. **So, one of the most important questions to be considered by a medical school is: will the student complete the course?**

Finally, medical schools are also looking for students who will contribute to the broad spectrum of university life. Those who do so are so much more likely to gain a wider experience of working and communicating with people from different backgrounds.

The admissions tutor's perspective

In deciding who will and who will not to be invited to study Medicine at their university, medical schools look to the views of their admissions tutors, the people who read the application submissions and who conduct the interviews.

And when reading hundreds of Personal Statements, so often the key considerations of the tutors are:

'Does this candidate have a sense of what they are going to get into by studying Medicine, and indeed by studying Medicine at this medical school?'

'Can I see this individual becoming a good practising doctor in a few years from now?'

Whilst it is likely that admissions tutors will be looking to see if you possess the personal qualities so often associated with doctors - qualities such as kindness, compassion, empathy, and curiosity - they are perhaps even more determined to see if you are always reliable, and that you can handle the physical, mental and emotional strains you will experience, firstly as a medical student and then as a professional practitioner.

Key message

Selection for medical school implies selection for the medical profession.

Medical schools want candidates with more than academic ability. They want to train the doctors of tomorrow.

Chapter 3

The essential contents of the Personal Statement

Your Personal Statement is your opportunity to describe in words:

a) The reasons why you are so keen to study Medicine, and at the universities to which you are submitting your applications

b) That even in advance of taking up your medical studies, you have already made a real commitment to this course of action by gaining relevant experience

c) That you have a good idea of, and are equipped to handle, the expectations, responsibilities, pressures and duties attached to the practice of medicine

d) That you are special, and possess attributes which will see you through your medical course and towards establishing your medical professional career

Let us take each of these themes above and look at them carefully.

Why medicine?

"What is medicine?

Medicine offers a broad range of careers from general practice to the specialties of hospital practice and to medical research. Medicine is an applied science, but it is equally about dealing sympathetically and effectively with individuals, whether they be patients or colleagues. Medicine increasingly poses difficult ethical dilemmas, and, above all, medicine is constantly and rapidly developing and providing a stimulating challenge to practitioners and medical scientists alike. "

Oxford University website
June 2007

Every would-be medical student has their own story as to how and why they came to make that academic - and career- choice. In your Personal Statement, it is vital that you explain **YOUR** own journey in **YOUR** own **unique** way. But you must present your story with real **conviction**.

In 2006, editors of the British Medical Journal asked three doctors who are responsible for some of the most inspiring medical textbooks to write upon the theme of 'Why medicine inspires me?' (BMJ Vol 333 23-30th Dec 2006 pgs 1320-1323. The following extracts are reproduced with permission from the BMJ Publishing Group). Their accounts are incredibly illuminating and written with great passion.

Here are some of their comments:

'As is hopefully true for all doctors, I am inspired by the opportunity to spend my professional lifetime trying to improve the health and welfare of humanity.

I always believed that no higher calling existed than to help individual patients.'

'I find it hard to look back and capture what initially inspired me to take up medicine, but I think that my aspirations are still the same. Medicine is a 'way of life' and combines that rather nebulous feeling of wanting to help and care with the more exact principles of science and logical thought. After all these years as a doctor, I still want to get out of bed and go to work in the mornings.'

'Doctors are at the top of the list of professions that the public thinks are worthy of "respect" and also are "most likely to tell the truth", and this makes me feel privileged to be a doctor.'

'There is no place for arrogance or self-satisfaction. I still relish a diagnostic conundrum that calls on all my faculties and training to tease it out. I have been fortunate to treat people from different ethnic groups with different cultures, beliefs and diseases. This has been a humbling experience but also educational and fascinating.'

'Medicine offers a huge variety of choices - clinical work, research, teaching, training and management - to name but a few. Medicine is currently undergoing many changes. The medical curriculum has changed almost beyond recognition since I was a student. More emphasis is placed on communication and clinical skills. The greatest joy is that simple "thank you" as the patient walks out of the door. Isn't it great?'

'Medicine is based on altruism, science, and human interest. Like most medical students, this is what attracted me and it still does. The aspirations are of excellent care, progress, and change. I find the continuing movement,

and certainty that we will know more, inspirational and energising. Medicine is remarkable in its clinical and scientific breadth and its fusion with other disciplines and interests. Much of medicine grows from basic biology, but medical research and practice is also linked to physics, chemistry, statistics, population science, sociology and politics. It is remarkable, for example, that new technical platforms allow quick identification of genetic patterns that in future may influence treatment given to individual patients and that this, in turn, will raise ethical and political issues for society at large.'

'Whatever interests and personality you have, there is probably an aspect of medicine to suit you. The diversity can be confusing for a student and young doctor thinking about a career. When I qualified I did not know what would be the best path to choose.'

'Teaching and training are essential components of medicine. Brilliant lectures and articles and new discoveries and ideas are great rejuvenators. Cancer medicine has been a constant source of inspiration. Few areas of medicine demand the same degree of technical expertise and human understanding. The constant development of new approaches is engrossing.'

Clearly, these accounts are written with the wisdom which comes after many years of medical experience. But the statements really do deserve careful consideration; they were written by doctors, to be read, very largely, by other doctors.

For example, look at the ways these authors describe their enthusiasm for medicine: in particular, note the use of words such as *'inspired'*, *'aspirations'*, *'relish'*, *'energising'*, *'engrossing'*.

Look also at their references to the challenges and uncertainties which accompany medical studies. For example, *'The diversity can be confusing for a student'* and *'When I qualified I did not know what would be the best path to choose'*.

When writing your own Personal Statement, you must write in your own style. However, you can be sure that admissions tutors are looking to see evidence of **enthusiasm** and careful **reflection** in your comments.

Why medicine at this university?

Before you begin to write your medical school Personal Statement you need to decide the medical schools to which you wish to apply. It is important that you consult a careers advisor and visit the medical schools yourself before making your final decision. This is a decision not to be taken lightly given the fact that you will be dedicating the next several years to studying there.

There are many factors to take into account when considering your choice, including:

- Would you prefer to study at a campus or city based medical school?

- Do you feel comfortable in the locality in which the medical school is set?

- Are you happy with the educational approaches taken by the medical schools under consideration? These do vary. For example, some courses concentrate on Problem Based Learning, a style of teaching which is based on the consideration of case studies, or scenarios, and the students presenting their findings in

> the context of achieving defined educational objectives.
> - When would you start interacting with patients?
> - What extracurricular activities are available?
> - Do you want to study close to your family home, or not?

Each medical school has a slightly different selection process so it is important that you also visit their website in order to obtain the necessary details. A list of websites for all medical schools in the UK can be viewed at

www.apply2medicine.co.uk/medical-schools

Your commitment to medical studies and a medical career

Consider the situation in which a Premier League football club is considering whether or not to offer a teenage boy, with aspirations to be a professional footballer, a position within the club's youth academy. You can be sure that in addition to their consideration of his football ability, the club's coaches will also be looking to see signs of a real commitment to a future career in the sport as demonstrated by, for example, his approach to diet, and his attitude to drinking and smoking. In short, the club will be keen to see evidence of personal investment in this career move. What is he keen to do; what is he prepared to give up?

The same applies in the consideration of medical school applications. The admissions tutors will be keen to find out how you spend your time outside the formal school curriculum.

For example, they may look to see if your Personal Statement contains evidence that

- You try to keep abreast of medical developments as they are reported in leading medical journals (for example, The Lancet, The BMJ) and the national newspapers, or

- You spend time at weekends supporting staff in a local hospice, care home or hospital.

Understanding the expectations, responsibilities and duties attached to the practice of medicine

The most authoritative description of the responsibilities and duties of doctors working in the United Kingdom is that issued by the General Medical Council (GMC), the body with which all medical practitioners in our country must become registered.

Presented overleaf is the statement from the GMC defining the duties of a doctor taken from 'Good Medical Practice', November 2006. **It is imperative that all applicants to medical school gain a full understanding of the GMC's requirements.**

The Duties of a Doctor registered with the General Medical Council

Patients must be able to trust doctors with their lives and health. To justify that trust you must show respect for human life.

And you must:

- Make the care of patients your first concern

- Protect and promote the health of patients and the public

- Provide a good standard of practice and care

  - Keep your professional knowledge and skills up to date

  - Recognise and work within the limits of your professional competence

  - Work with colleagues in the ways that best serve patients' interests

- Treat patients as individuals and respect their dignity

  - Treat patients politely and considerately

  - Respect patients' right to confidentiality

- Work in partnership with patients

  - Listen to patients and respond to their concerns and preferences

  - Give patients the information they want and in a way they can understand

---

- – Respect patients' right to reach decisions with you about their treatment and care

- – Support patients in caring for themselves to improve and maintain their health

- • Be honest and trustworthy

- – Act without delay if you have good reason to believe that you or a colleague may be putting patients at risk

- – Never discriminate unfairly against patients or colleagues

- – Never abuse your patients' trust in you or the public's trust in the profession

You are personally accountable for your professional practice and must always be prepared to justify your decisions and actions.

Accordingly, by drawing upon your experiences in life, especially your work experience, it is vital that you use your Personal Statement to convince the admissions tutors that you are able to:

- • Engage appropriately with ill or disabled people, and

- • Listen to them and to support them, and

- • Work effectively as a member of a team.

Remember, *"There is no place for arrogance or self-satisfaction"* and that setting a course upon becoming a doctor is a *"humbling experience"*.

It is also important that you indicate your understanding of the physical and emotional demands placed upon medical students and doctors.

It is indeed a *"way of life"*: doctors are so often seen as role models for society.

Finally, by all means indicate where your specific medical career interests might presently lie BUT also understand that your views may well change in the light of your medical education and clinical experiences.

Show them you are special

When considering the Personal Statements of applicants to medical schools, the admissions tutors will also be asking themselves:

- *Has this applicant really thought things through?*

- *Do we want to meet this candidate at interview?*

- *Do we see them enjoying and completing their studies, well on their way to becoming a good doctor?*

- *Will it be good for the university to have this candidate around?*

Your Personal Statement is your opportunity to influence the tutors towards saying 'Yes' in response to each of these questions as they apply to you!

So, it is important that you write in a way that depicts the enthusiasm, keenness – and indeed, **passion-** you have for your chosen academic choice.

Phrases such as 'I am *quite* interested in studying Medicine' or 'I really *think* that Medicine is the right course for me' are to be avoided; they are so unconvincing! And if you have received special commendations or prizes, write about them in a way that shows how they reinforce your decision to study Medicine.

For example, if you became Head Pupil at your school, this clearly shows the strength of the teachers' regard for your leadership qualities, and your ability to act as a role model for other pupils. So, elaborate upon those themes! Equally, if you worked effectively as part of a team raising money for your school's charity you could describe how this experience improved your teamwork and communication skills.

It is vitally important when referring to your experiences in your Personal Statement to clearly state how these have developed in you the qualities that are required of a medical student and future doctor.

However, before you submit your final statement, you would also do well to talk about your 'special' qualities to your referee. Some comments are simply more effectively made by another person and it is important that your Reference fully supports your application to medical school.

Key message

It is vital that you use your medical school Personal Statement to convince the admissions tutors that you have really considered the implications of studying Medicine AND that you know that it is right for you.

Chapter 4

Medical School applications: The Myths

During our experience in supporting students in their applications to medical schools, we have come across many misunderstandings. Here are some which arise time after time!

1. **Medical schools are keen to meet students whose key motivation for wishing to become a doctor is due to a parent being a doctor.**

No. Clearly, the fact that one of your parents is a doctor may very significantly account for your keen interest in studying Medicine. However, this is simply not sufficient justification for your decision to embark upon a medical career. Admissions tutors will be looking to see how you have carefully considered your career options, and how you have confirmed your final choice by gaining appropriate experience.

2. **It is easier to get into medical school if your parent is a doctor.**

This is not true. Again, if your parent is a doctor it is certainly easier to gain an insight into the world of medicine. However, medical schools are interested in each individual applicant and in the steps they have undertaken to confirm that they have the right qualities for a future medical career.

3. Medical schools are much more likely to take students from private schools.

This is simply not true – medical schools look to offer places to the best candidates regardless of whether they attended a private or state school. Your suitability for gaining an interview and subsequent place will be determined by the quality of your university application, including particularly the effort that you have placed in preparing your Personal Statement. Remember, together with your predicted grades, it is predominantly the strength of your Personal Statement and your Reference that will determine whether you are invited to attend an interview or not.

4. I am the first person to ever apply to medical school from my school, therefore I don't stand a chance of getting in.

This is not true and a common misconception. Simply because you may be the first person from your school or college to apply to study Medicine does not mean that your chances are reduced. Successful candidates are those who have invested time and effort in preparing their applications, and who have ensured that their referees became aware of their keen intentions to study Medicine.

5. I must achieve all A grades in my GCSEs and my A-levels to get into medical school.

This is not necessarily true and depends on the particular medical school and its entry requirements. It is therefore important that you carefully study the admissions criteria of the medical schools to which you intend to apply.

6. Despite my greatest efforts I have been unable to secure work experience in a medical setting therefore I will not be able to apply to medical school.

Although for some people it may be difficult to secure work experience within a hospital or general practice surgery, there are many other options open to you that will enable you to gain first hand experience of working with ill or disabled people. These include working:

- At a care or nursing home
- In a hospice
- Within a voluntary organisation, such as St John's Ambulance or The Samaritans
- With support groups for the disabled

Remember, your work experience is crucial in enabling you to obtain first hand experience of working with, and helping to improve the quality of life of, ill or disabled people, and confirming that you have what it takes to follow this through and establish a medical career.

7. Scoring well in my examinations is the only thing I need to do to get into medical school.

Not true at all. Yes, successful applicants to medical schools will obtain excellent academic results; however, it is vital that they also demonstrate that they have the qualities required of a good doctor. Think back to your own experiences when you were treated by a doctor: what special qualities made them stand out? Some of these include:

- Having a real desire to help people
- Being able to communicate clearly
- Understanding the importance of effective team working and leadership skills
- Being empathic and honest
- Recognising the importance of adopting a conscientious and highly motivated approach

8. When describing your work experience you should not refer to non-medical experience.

It is important to refer to your medical and your non-medical experiences to demonstrate how these have helped to equip you in your forthcoming studies, and beyond! For example, someone describing that they had led a mountaineering expedition would clearly demonstrate their strong leadership and team working skills.

9. **My Personal Statement must be exactly 4,000 characters or I will be penalised.**

Obviously, the more relevant information you include within the allowed space then the more fully you will be able to tell the admissions tutors about yourself and why you should be offered a place at their medical school. However, it really is about quality not quantity, so do not attempt to pad out your Personal Statement with irrelevant facts that do not add any value to your application or, worse still, weaken it.

10. **The sooner I submit my Personal Statement before the deadline the better my chances of success.**

This is another common misconception. The only real advantage of submitting your medical school application as early as possible is that it will reduce your stress levels and enable you to concentrate on your studies. Despite what is commonly perceived, submitting your application earlier rather than later will not mean that you stand a better chance of your application progressing simply because it is at the top of the admission tutor's pile!

11. **If I select two other course choices in addition to Medicine I will reduce my chances.**

Admissions tutors will not think that you are less committed to studying Medicine if you list two other courses in addition to the four medical school applications you have submitted. Indeed, unless the courses you have selected are at the same university, the Data Protection Act precludes admissions tutors the ability to identify your other applications.

However, it is important that your Personal Statement is 100% tailored to your application to study Medicine and does not contain reference to other non-medical courses.

Key message

Your Personal Statement is your opportunity to justify to the admissions tutors why YOU, as a UNIQUE INDIVIDUAL, should be accepted to medical school in the first step of a medical career.

Chapter 5

Preparing your Personal Statement

Check the key questions

The first step in preparing your Personal Statement is to take a good look at yourself- your personality, your strengths and your achievements. Then take a blank piece of paper and write down where you stand with regard to the key questions set out below. It is almost certain that you will not be able to touch upon each and every topic covered by these questions in your final Personal Statement. However, it will be helpful for you to consider each question; you can then decide which areas you are keen to include and which ones you are content to discard.

You might also find it valuable to have to hand the following when considering the key questions below:

- The list of 'Duties of a doctor registered with the General Medical Council' (pages 18 to 19)

- The guiding principles for the admission of medical students formulated by the Council of Heads of Medical Schools (pages 7 to 9) and

- The quotations relating to 'Why medicine inspires me' (pages 12 to 14)

But please note: it is extremely important that when it comes to writing your Personal Statement, you create your own expressions and phrases. Your Personal Statement has to be written uniquely in your style - about you!

Key questions:

- When and why did you begin to be interested in Medicine?

- Why do you want to study Medicine? Are you sure you want to be a doctor? Why do you want to be a doctor rather than, for example, a nurse, or a physiotherapist? Or a lawyer?

- Why are you so keen to study Medicine at this particular university?

- What kind of person are you? Which aspects of your personality equip you well for medical studies and a career in medicine?

- What are your strengths and weaknesses? What are your strengths and weaknesses according to others, such as your parents, your friends, your teachers? What special talents do you have which could be of real value within a medical career?

- What work experience have you had which has given you a special insight into life as a medical student or as a doctor?

- What else have you done, or has happened to you, which has provided excellent learning experiences or drawn upon your special personal qualities, such as compassion, tenacity, empathy?

- What awards or prizes (academic and non-academic) have you received? What do these tell people about you?
- What are your keen interests outside academic studies?
- What do you see yourself doing in 5 or 10 years time.

Drafting a structure

Three important sections

When complete, an effective Personal Statement will comprise three key sections: your 'Introduction', a 'Conclusion', and between these two sections will lie those paragraphs comprising the 'Main Body' of the Personal Statement.

It is helpful to sketch onto a piece of blank paper three boxes; one labelled 'Introduction', one labelled 'Conclusion' and, lying between those two boxes, one labelled 'Main Body'.

Now start mapping some draft comments to each of the three sections.

The Introduction

The aim of the Introduction is to catch the attention of the reader, namely the admissions tutor. So, try and compose a statement which really grabs the reader's attention and enables you to stand out from the crowd!

The Main Body of the Personal Statement

The Main Body of your Personal Statement is the section in which you build upon your Introduction and describe:

- Why you have decided to study Medicine
- The steps you have taken in making a real commitment to study Medicine
- That you have a real sense of what medical studies and a subsequent medical career entail
- Aspects of yourself which especially equip you for this course of action

It is in this section that you will refer to:

- Your work experience, and the relevant insights it has given you towards confirming that studying Medicine is right for you
- The steps you have taken in furthering your interest in Medicine and medical matters
- The topics which you look forward to studying most
- Your experience of teamwork, leadership and responsibility, reliability and tenacity
- Your thoughts upon what direction your medical career might take, always recognising that this might change in the light of experience at medical school.

The Conclusion

It is vitally important to draw your Personal Statement to a close, and reaffirm that you are someone who will flourish academically and socially at medical school, and that you are well equipped to handle the stresses and strains associated with medical studies. The 'Conclusion' paragraph is not the time to introduce any new themes. However, not to present a concise, summary comment would be a real error of judgement.

Writing and improving your Personal Statement

In formulating the contents of each of the key sections (Introduction; Main Body; Conclusion) of your Personal Statement, it is important that you focus upon the following questions:

- Does each of your sections **-especially the Introduction,** and your Personal Statement as a whole have **real impact upon the reader?**

- Is the punctuation correct?

- Is the flow of your language appealing, non-repetitive and easy to follow?

- Is there a logical and coherent balance to the Personal Statement?

- Are all your statements absolutely honest and accurate? Remember! Anything you refer to in your Personal Statement may be the subject of questions at any subsequent interviews. Admissions tutors are very skilled at identifying situations when candidates have made exaggerated claims!

- Will the reader conclude that you are indeed 'special'? Is it truly about you?

And finally:

- **Have you concentrated on justifying and substantiating your comments?**

The admissions tutors will consider everything that you include in your Personal Statement to help them decide whether or not to offer you the opportunity to study Medicine at their university. It is not enough to write, for example: *'I want to study Medicine because Biology is my strongest subject, academically.'* To excel in a specific academic subject is simply not sufficient justification for seeking to make a career within medicine and all that it entails.

Look again at this statement from the quotations presented earlier in Chapter 3:

'I find it hard to look back and capture what initially inspired me to take up medicine, but I think that my aspirations are still the same. Medicine is a 'way of life' and combines that rather nebulous feeling of wanting to help and care with the more exact principles of science and logical thought.'

This writer provides clear evidence that it was the combination of their joy in scientific intellectual stimulation AND the opportunity to reach out and support others that inspired them to study Medicine and develop a medical career.

You must maintain your own focus upon justifying and substantiating your comments throughout your entire Personal Statement.

Key Message

You need time to write your Personal Statement, do not rush.

Prepare a first DRAFT, containing an Introduction, a Main Body and a Conclusion.

Chapter 6

From 'Draft' to 'Refined'; enhancing your Personal Statement

One way by which we can illustrate the importance of focusing upon the key principles which govern the preparation of an effective, compelling Personal Statement is to consider a fictitious example, initially in its first 'draft' form, and then looking at it after some refinement. The critique which follows should not be interpreted as 'definitive', or 'state of the art'. And certainly, there is no such thing as the perfect Personal Statement. However, we hope that by using this scenario - moving from a 'draft' to a 'refined' version - we can bring the whole process to life!

Fictitious Personal Statement: 'Draft' version

I have always been fascinated by medicine so I would really like the chance to study it at university. My father and grandfather are both respected doctors and my ambition is to hold a similarly highly regarded position in the community.

I have thoroughly enjoyed studying A levels in Biology, Physics and Chemistry and I also enjoy reading other books about developments in science and I believe I will enjoy studying medicine at University. To explore the subject further I have been to the Med-Link conference at Manchester University in 2005 and Med-Sim at Nottingham University in 2006.

I have also taken on some work experience in a range of medical areas. I started in 2003 working at Hope House near Reading, which is a residential school for disabled children. I worked there every Wednesday and Saturday afternoon for two years during term-time. Last summer, I went with a group to Ireland for a week to work in a hospice as a volunteer looking after some of the patients there. This was a very demanding experience but it did not discourage me, rather it was one of the most amazing experiences of my life and I plan to return next year. I have also recently started a permanent position as a ward volunteer at Reading District General Hospital. I have also discussed my future career with family members who work in medicine, and I am confident that I am well suited to this career.

I am a keen member of the school science club and I am also captain of the football team, which has won several local tournaments. Playing football and supporting my favourite team, Arsenal, at matches both home and away has given me the chance to meet new people and develop skills in teamworking and leadership. I have also been involved in other extra curricular activities through completing the Duke of Edinbrugh silver award. I am also a senior prefect. Art is another hobby of mine, and I like to visit various art galleries in my holidays. I love travelling and I have been to Canada, the USA, France, Italy and Spain. For this reason, I jumped at the chance of a gap year, and I will be working in Britain for six months before I set off travelling.

Character Count: 2,153

Fictitious Personal Statement: 'Refined' version

A career in medicine appeals to me as it combines my enjoyment of science with my desire to contribute towards improving the health and well being of people. As several of my relatives are doctors I have benefited from discussions with them about the realities of a medical career, highlighting both the challenges and the rewards.

At school I have found the practical elements of my science subjects particularly fascinating; for example, learning how to use new equipment and materials during experiments. Within Biology I have especially enjoyed learning about the functions of the human body and how different organs behave in health and in disease. Keeping up to date with advances and breakthroughs in medical science is another keen interest of mine, and I regularly read journals such as New Scientist and the BMJ. As a member of the school science club I always look forward to the opportunity to discuss relevant current issues. For example, we had a lively debate about the recent MRSA problems and what might be done to improve the situation; recently, I gave a short presentation on human stem cell cloning. I am really looking forward to learning more about the ethical issues relating to medical advances during my degree course. Attending the Medlink and Medsim conferences was a valuable way to raise my awareness of what training and a career in medicine will involve, including the need for commitment to the continual updating of my skills and knowledge.

A long-term part time placement at a residential school for disabled children introduced me to the basics of providing personal care and the need for a sensitive and empathic approach when talking to patients and their families. This was useful experience for a subsequent position at a hospice in Ireland during which my duties were to befriend and chat to elderly patients. Here I learnt from the nurses about issues such as patient confidentiality and autonomy. My time at the hospice was particularly intense as many of the patients were suffering from mental illnesses associated with cancer. However, I felt inspired by the caring approaches shown by the staff and overall the experience reinforced my commitment towards contributing to this field. Recently, I have obtained a weekend position as a ward volunteer at my local general hospital. This has been invaluable in giving me an understanding of how a hospital is run and the functions of the different members of a medical team. My duties so far have involved helping to serve meals, assisting with the personal care of the more mobile patients, and helping with clerical duties in the ward reception area.

In my leisure time I enjoy sport, particularly tennis and football. Captaining my school football team, which has won several local tournaments, has hugely helped me in developing strengths in leadership and teamwork. Completing the Duke of Edinburgh silver award gave me the opportunity to learn a range of new skills, including playing the piano and organising fund raising events. As a senior prefect I am responsible for organising the duties of other prefects; I also assist teachers in supervising lower school pupils at mealtimes and breaktimes. My gap year-during which I intend to travel around South East Asia - will help equip me to live independently and prepare me for the transition between home and university life. Working in a supermarket for six months before leaving will enable me to save the money required and I am confident that a year out of education will be a maturing experience for me.

In conclusion, I am a self-motivated, enthusiastic and determined student who enjoys close interaction with people. I feel prepared for the demands and challenges that a medical career entails. I look forward to the opportunity to read Medicine, in order both to fulfil my ambition of becoming a doctor and to serve the community.

Character Count: 3,894

Moving from 'Draft' to 'Refined': Improving your Personal Statement

The following analysis aims to help you to create an engaging Personal Statement by looking at ways the above 'Draft' statement was refined. By considering the 'Draft' and 'Refined' paragraphs side by side, important principles can be highlighted.

Paragraph One: Draft

'I have always been fascinated by medicine so I would really like the chance to study it at university. My father and grandfather are both respected doctors and my ambition is to hold a similarly highly regarded position in the community.'

Paragraph One: Refined

'A career in medicine appeals to me as it combines my enjoyment of science with my desire to contribute towards improving the health and well being of people.

As several of my relatives are doctors, I have benefited from discussions with them about the realities of a medical career, highlighting both the challenges and the rewards.'

Paragraph One: Draft

The opening sentence is not particularly attention grabbing and does not give the admissions tutors any information beyond that the applicant wants to study Medicine; the admissions panel will have assumed this to be the case anyway.

'I would really like the chance' is not language depicting a passionate interest in a subject area.

Beware of claiming to have *'always'* been interested in medicine. Even if you did want to be a doctor at the age of three, you would not at that point have had the ability to make an informed decision on the subject. It can sound naïve to imply that you are applying to study a subject because it was your childhood dream. The tutors are looking to see if your choice is based upon careful, mature consideration.

The use of the phrase *'my ambition is to hold a ... highly regarded position in the community'* smacks somewhat of a self-seeking motivation. Remember that having a relative or family friend in the medical profession does not in itself improve the applicant's chances of gaining an interview. **If the applicant feels they have benefited from having frequent contact with a practising doctor, it is important that they show they have made use of this opportunity to learn more about the medical career.**

Paragraph One: Refined

By beginning the Personal Statement with a clear and well reasoned explanation of their reason for applying, the candidate now makes a bold and engaging opening sentence and also indicates that they have considered their career choices carefully. This paragraph, therefore, really has become an 'Introduction' to the rest of the Personal Statement.

The influence of family members who are doctors is discussed and the applicant refers to the value gained from this personal contact. This does suggest that they are well informed about life as a doctor and therefore may well be the type of person to make the most of opportunities around them.

• • • • • •

Paragraph Two: Draft

'I have thoroughly enjoyed studying A levels in Biology, Physics and Chemistry and I also enjoy reading other books about developments in science and I believe I will enjoy studying medicine at University. To explore the subject further I have been to the Med-Link conference at Manchester University in 2005 and Med-Sim at Nottingham University in 2006.'

Paragraph Two: Refined

'At school I have found the practical elements of my science subjects particularly fascinating; for example, learning how to use new equipment and materials during experiments. Within Biology I have especially enjoyed learning about the functions of the human body and how different organs behave in health and in disease. Keeping up to date with advances and breakthroughs in medical science is another keen interest of mine, and I regularly read journals such as New Scientist and the BMJ. As a member of the school science club I always look forward to the opportunity

---

to discuss relevant current issues. For example, we had a lively debate about the recent MRSA problems and what might be done to improve the situation; recently, I gave a short presentation on human stem cell cloning. I am really looking forward to learning more about the ethical issues relating to medical advances during my degree course. Attending the Medlink and Medsim conferences was a valuable way to raise my awareness of what training and a career in medicine will involve, including the need for commitment to the continual updating of my skills and knowledge.'

Paragraph Two: Draft

Describing the A-level subjects which you are studying, information which is picked up elsewhere on your application, simply wastes valuable word space. Although the applicant asserts that they enjoy science, no specific examples are presented in substantiation of that comment. Always ensure that you assign a capital letter to the name of the university course. However, 'university' when used in the general way carries no capital letter. So, *'studying medicine at University'* should read *'studying Medicine at university'*. (Note: It <u>is</u> appropriate for the candidate to provide the capital letters in the specific phrases *'Manchester University'* and *'Nottingham University.'*)

The tone of the paragraph is not enthusiastic: for example, the phrase *'I believe I will enjoy studying medicine at University'* lacks conviction. Remember also that the majority of your fellow applicants will have taken similar subjects at A-level and will be predicted similar grades. Coming early in the 'Main Body' of the Personal

Statement, this paragraph provides your opportunity to describe what particularly enthuses **You** and what **You** especially enjoy about the learning process. The admissions tutors will be looking for people who are enthusiastic about the prospect of studying Medicine at their university for several years, as well as looking forward to practising as a doctor later. Although the applicant writes that they like books relating to science, not a single example is cited.

The applicant then states that they have attended Medsim and Medlink conferences but does not explain what they learnt or gained from the experience. Again, remember that many of your fellow applicants will have attended similar conferences; it is up to you to show how this experience has made you a stronger candidate. It is also important not to waste your word limit giving too much irrelevant detail. For example, there is no real need to refer to the location of the conferences you have attended.

Some of the phrases are repetitive: the word '*I*' is used five times in less than five lines of text; the words '*enjoyed*' and '*enjoy*' three times.

Overall, this paragraph adds very little to the Personal Statement and misses an opportunity to show how the applicant has prepared themselves for the academic rigour required in studying for a medical degree.

Paragraph Two: Refined

This version provides much greater detail about what the applicant has learnt from their academic experience over the last couple of years. **By describing elements of the subjects which they enjoy, the candidate now**

highlights their skills in, and their enthusiasm for, practical aspects of science as well as demonstrating an awareness of how their A-level subjects have helped them in preparation for degree level study.

By referring to specific relevant journals and current issues in medicine, the applicant now shows that they are reading outside the school curriculum and provides examples of specific educational areas of interest; their Personal Statement now demonstrates that they have invested some of their own time in support of their commitment to studying Medicine.

Describing what has been gained from the Medlink and Medsim conferences has the same impact. The statements regarding the science club have been moved to this paragraph as they read more fluently and relevantly: they provide good evidence that the candidate has gained valuable experience in broader academic skills, such as conducting self-directed research and in preparing and delivering presentations.

(But remember: referring to, for example, The BMJ, provides an open invitation to any interviewer to ask you questions such as 'Tell me about a recent article you have read which has impressed you in some way'. So, make sure you mean exactly what you say in your Personal Statement – and that you do your preparation for interview in that light!!)

● ● ● ● ● ●

Paragraph Three: Draft

'I have also taken on some work experience in a range of medical areas. I started in 2003 working at Hope House near Reading, which is a residential school for disabled children. I worked there every Wednesday and Saturday afternoon for two years during term-time. Last summer, I went with a group to Ireland for a week to work in a hospice as a volunteer looking after some of the patients there. This was a very demanding experience but it did not discourage me, rather it was one of the most amazing experiences of my life and I plan to return next year. I have also recently started a permanent position as a ward volunteer at Reading District General Hospital. I have also discussed my future career with family members who work in medicine, and I am confident that I am well suited to this career.'

Paragraph Three: Refined

'A long-term part time placement at a residential school for disabled children introduced me to the basics of providing personal care and the need for a sensitive and empathic approach when talking to patients and their families. This was useful experience for a subsequent position at a hospice in Ireland during which my duties were to befriend and chat to elderly patients. Here I learnt from the nurses about issues such as patient confidentiality and autonomy. My time at the hospice was particularly intense as many of the patients were suffering from mental illnesses associated with cancer. However, I felt inspired by the caring approaches shown by the staff and overall the experience reinforced my

commitment towards contributing to this field. Recently, I have obtained a weekend position as a ward volunteer at my local general hospital. This has been invaluable in giving me an understanding of how a hospital is run and the functions of the different members of a medical team. My duties so far have involved helping to serve meals, assisting with the personal care of the more mobile patients, and helping with clerical duties in the ward reception area.

Paragraph Three: Draft

Although the applicant refers to areas of work experience which may well have been extremely helpful when considering whether or not to study Medicine, there is no reflection upon exactly how those experiences helped them to make that decision.

The opening phrase, *'I have also taken on some work experience'* sounds apologetic and wholly lacks enthusiasm. Equally, the *'range of medical areas'* begs the (unanswered) question- exactly which areas? And although describing working in a hospice in Ireland as *'one of the most amazing experiences of my life'* there is absolutely no comment upon why that was the case!

There is also too much space wasted with irrelevant details such as precise times, names and locations. Such details add nothing to the strength of the application. The phrase *'I am confident that I am well suited to this career'* would be better placed within a concluding paragraph.

The phrase *'I have also'* is used three times. The word *'I'* is used nine times!

Paragraph Three: Refined

The refined version now shows the candidate reflecting upon their work as a volunteer to highlight the experience gained in so many aspects of medical professional work – personal care, empathy, ethical issues, teamwork - and how it has helped them to decide on a career in medicine. Their placement in Ireland clearly was a remarkable experience and served to remind them also of the demands placed upon medical staff when carrying out their day-to-day duties.

Note again:

Because the candidate has introduced topics such as *'patient confidentiality'* and *'autonomy'* it would be vital that they obtain a full understanding of their meaning and significance before any interview. By referring to a special interest in the field of mental illness, a similar need for careful interview preparation also applies.

Perhaps the most important aspect of your Personal Statement is the way in which you describe the insights you have gained from your work experience – and indeed how those insights have further encouraged you to pursue a medical career.

• • • • • •

Paragraph Four: Draft

'I am a keen member of the school science club and I am also captain of the football team, which has won several local tournaments. Playing football and supporting my favourite team, Arsenal, at matches both home and away has given me the chance to meet new people and develop skills in teamworking and leadership. I have also been involved in other extra curricular activities through completing the Duke of Edinbrugh silver award. I am also a senior prefect. Art is another hobby of mine, and I like to visit various art galleries in my holidays. I love travelling and I have been to Canada, the USA, France, Italy and Spain. For this reason, I jumped at the chance of a gap year, and I will be working in Britain for six months before I set off travelling.'

Paragraph Four: Refined

'In my leisure time I enjoy sport, particularly tennis and football. Captaining my school football team, which has won several local tournaments, has hugely helped me in developing strengths in leadership and teamwork. Completing the Duke of Edinburgh silver award gave me the opportunity to learn a range of new skills, including playing the piano and organising fund raising events. As a senior prefect I am responsible for organising the duties of other prefects; I also assist teachers in supervising lower school pupils at mealtimes and breaktimes. My gap year- during which I intend to travel around South East Asia- will help equip me to live independently and prepare me for the transition

> between home and university life. Working in a supermarket for six months before leaving will enable me to save the money required and I am confident that a year out of education will be a maturing experience for me.'

Paragraph Four: Draft

'Edinbrugh' is an incorrect spelling of the Scottish capital city: the admissions tutors will take a dim view of this example of carelessness! The text reads uninterestingly and the applicant simply lists areas of interest with almost no shades of emphasis or significance- apart from their keenness (*'jumped at'*) to take the opportunity of a year away from academic studies!

The applicant fails entirely to detail how their role as captain of the school football team gives them insights into teamworking and leadership, nor do they touch upon the learning value attached to their responsibilities as a senior prefect.

It is hard to see how supporting Arsenal at matches *'home and away'* equips a candidate for medical studies; however, it does indicate how this applicant spends some of their recreational time, inviting a comparison between this and how they invest time in furthering their commitment to a medical career.

They also completely fail to describe the relevance, if any, of their trips to several foreign countries or art galleries.

The word *'I'* is used ten times.

Paragraph Four: Refined

The points raised about recreational interests and hobbies now focus so much more upon the relevance these pursuits have to the application itself. Details are given as to how being the captain of the football team and involvement in the Duke of Edinburgh award has helped them become a well-rounded person. Some responsibilities of being a senior prefect are given and the paragraph points to the contributions the student may make to the university community. In their reference to the gap year, they indicate that they have planned a structured year in preparation for life at medical school.

• • • • • •

Concluding Paragraph

The 'draft' Personal Statement ends by specifically referring, for the first time, to the theme of the gap year.

The opportunity is not taken to sum up key messages in a final, concluding comment.

Concluding Paragraph: Refined

'In conclusion, I am a self-motivated, enthusiastic and determined student who enjoys close interaction with people. I feel prepared for the demands and challenges that a medical career entails. I look forward to the opportunity to read Medicine, in order both to fulfil my ambition of becoming a doctor and to serve the community.

Concluding Paragraph: Draft

The candidate has completely failed to take the opportunity to make a final, summary comment. It is as if their entire Personal Statement is left 'hanging in the air'.

Concluding Paragraph: Refined

The applicant provides a final summary of their personal qualities aimed at convincing the reader of the sincerity of their application. The closing phrase *'to serve the community'* suggests some understanding of the importance of humility.

Key message

The 'Draft' and 'Refined' versions of this fictitious example are presented in order to illustrate the principles underpinning the preparation of a compelling Personal Statement.

<u>YOUR</u> Personal Statement must describe <u>YOU</u>; <u>YOUR</u> personal qualities, <u>YOUR</u> enthusiasms, <u>YOUR</u> strengths.

Make sure the material you present in your Personal Statement really does convince the reader that you have a very good idea of what you are getting into, that studying Medicine is right for you, <u>AND</u> that you are right for the medical profession.

Chapter 7

Proofreading your Personal Statement

When you believe that you are ready to submit your Personal Statement, **DON'T** until you are sure you are happy with its final format. It is also very useful to ask other people to read through your final version; it is amazing how helpful it is to obtain the viewpoint from 'a fresh pair of eyes'. For example, it may be very useful to receive the comments from an English teacher, especially with regard to your punctuation and writing style. Equally, there may be people you met during your work experience who would be pleased to help you in this way. BUT, remember that at the end of the day it is **YOUR** Personal Statement and if you feel passionate about an issue to the point that you are determined to include it, then do so!

Final checklist:

- Do you have a punchy and attention grabbing introduction?

- Do you come over as passionate about studying Medicine?

- Do you indicate that you have given serious practical consideration to the implications of establishing a medical career for **You?**

- Do you describe how your academic and extra-curricular activities have helped you to make this choice?

- Is every piece of information you provide clearly relevant to your application to study Medicine?

- Is your Personal Statement arranged in paragraphs? Is it balanced? Does it flow?

- Does your Personal Statement contain a concluding paragraph?

- Check all spelling and all punctuation

Submitting your medical school application

The majority of medical school applications are submitted electronically. Your Personal Statement needs to be typed up electronically and must not exceed 47 lines and 4,000 characters (~580-620 words. 12 Times New Roman).

If you are applying through your school or college, you will be provided with directions as to how to proceed. Those applying independently, such as graduates or mature students, can register directly on the UCAS website.

For more information visit www.ucas.com.

Key message
Keep looking for ways to IMPROVE upon your draft effort.
Invite others to PROOFREAD your statement before you finally submit it.

Chapter 8

Medical School Personal Statement: Things to avoid

This guide has focussed upon helping you how to draft, structure, refine, and proofread your Personal Statement.

Here is a list of some things to avoid!

- Rushing the preparation of your Personal Statement- you will need plenty of time to write it!

- Needlessly repeating information that is contained in other parts of your application

- Relying on a spell checking function – check it yourself; use a dictionary

- Dishonesty, or deliberately misleading the reader

- Using any word or phrase the meaning of which you are uncertain

- Trying to be funny. Just play it straight

- Drawing attention to any weakness, unless you have learnt from it, handled it, and become a more complete person

- Including comments which criticise others or casting yourself in a favourable light in comparison to others

- Simply listing achievements or interests; every comment must be relevant.

  Lists make for dry reading!

- Disjointed statements. Readers do not like having to flick backwards and forwards when trying to understand your comments

- Overuse of the 'I' word

- Lack of structure; lack of paragraphs

- Not proofreading your statement – ask your teachers, friends and family to help you in this regard. But remember that it is **your** personal statement!

Two final points:

Firstly, always make sure that your Personal Statement really is unique to you.

Secondly, make sure you keep a copy. You can be sure that if you are called for interview, panel members are almost certain to question you specifically upon some of the comments you have made. For you to say 'Oh, I forgot I wrote that' would give an incredibly bleak impression!

Chapter 9

Closing Thoughts

The aim of this guide is to provide you with a good idea of what should be included in your Personal Statement for application to medical schools in the UK. Our hope is that by following the principles and steps contained in this guide you will be able to compose a well-structured and effective Personal Statement.

In addition to this guide the Apply2Medicine website (www.apply2medicine.co.uk) contains lots of free resources, including details upon latest hot topics in the medical world, to help you prepare your application to medical school.

Apply2Medicine also offer a range of advisory services to help you to improve your Personal Statement and prepare for interview. All you need to do is to contact us at:

www.apply2medicine.co.uk/contact-us

0800 612 1135

We strongly recommend that you do seek more information from medical school websites and advice from staff at the medical school you wish to attend to ensure that your Personal Statement contains the information that they request.

From both Tony and Matt, we would like to wish you every success in securing your place at medical school.

Good Luck!!

Appendix

Valuable websites:

Universities and Colleges Admissions Service

www.ucas.com

Oxford Medical School

www.medsci.ox.ac.uk

General Medical Council

www.gmc-uk.org

Council of Medical School Heads

www.chms.ac.uk

Entrance Examinations

www.ukcat.ac.uk

www.bmat.org.uk

Apply2Medicine

www.apply2medicine.co.uk

Other books in the Apply2Medicine range available at www.apply2medicine.co.uk

'Your Medical School Interview: The Apply2Medicine Guide'

'Your Medical School Interview: The Apply2Medicine Guide' sets out the principles for success. The book highlights the importance of preparation – 'Your Homework' – and provides a framework through which you can effectively handle any question from the interview panel.

Testimonials from previous prospective medical students

The medicine examples Apply2Medicine provided me with were excellent. Together with the writing guide I was able to write a Personal Statement which was far better than I could have hoped

JK, London

I would like to thank you again for your help… I am really happy that I have chosen your service. I cannot begin to tell you how much I appreciated all the work you've done with me on my med school statement… I feel very lucky to have found your company. Thanks again and take care!

PV, Bournemouth

Thank you very much for this. I have been really impressed with your responsiveness and professionalism and WILL recommend you to others!

SG, Devon

Thanks a lot for providing such wonderful and prompt support. Without your help, I would not have been able to write my statement in such an amazing way. Thanks a lot again.

DI, Stevenage